INTERGENERATIONAL RELATIONSHIPS

Building Bonds Across Generations

John Dollar

Copyright © 2023

by

John dollar

Table Of Content

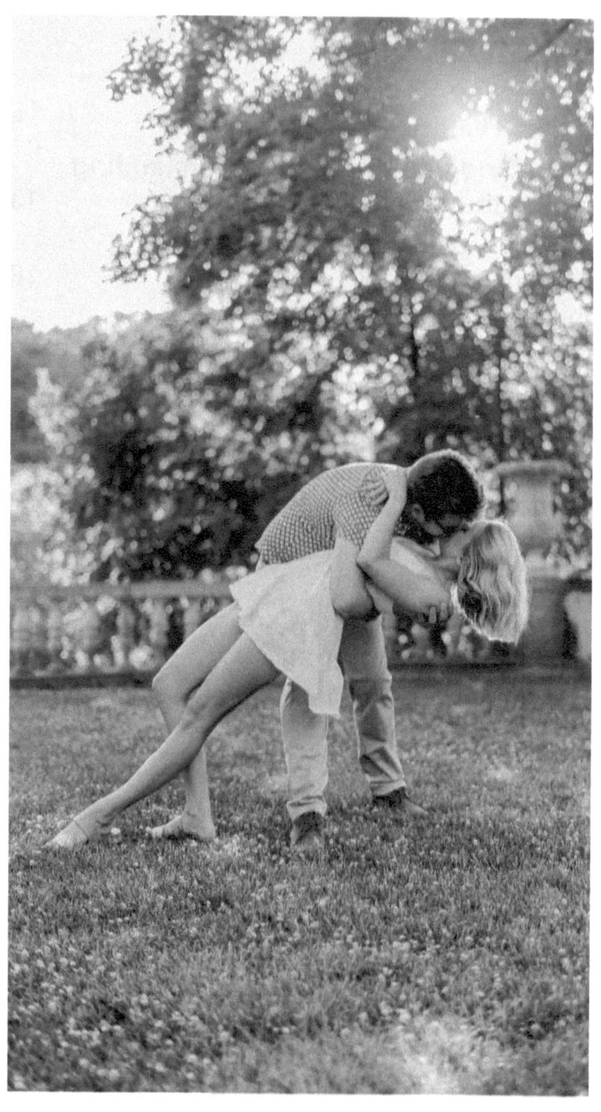

INTRODUCTION

In the quaint town of Eldridge, where time seemed to pass at its own leisurely pace, lived an unlikely couple bound together by threads of intergenerational connection. At one end stood Olivia, a spirited 25-year-old girl with dreams as wide as the sky, and at the other stood Mr. Harold, an 80-year-old widower whose eyes held the wisdom of countless yesterdays.

Their paths crossed one sunny afternoon at a local community center where Olivia volunteered to organize events for the elderly. Mr. Harold, a regular visitor, was initially skeptical of the young volunteers who moved around. But when he noticed Olivia's genuine smile and enthusiasm, something sparked his curiosity about the world outside his routine.

As the weeks turned into months, Olivia and Mr. Harold's friendship blossomed. They began spending afternoons together, exchanging stories that bridged the gap between their generations. With eyes sparkling like constellations, Olivia painted a vivid picture of the digital age where information flowed like a river and connections spanned the globe. Mr. Harold, in turn, unfolded the pages of history with stories from the days when handwritten letters were loved and face-to-face conversations were an art.

Eldridge Park became their favorite hangout, a timeless haven where the laughter of children echoed alongside the rustling of leaves. Under a wise old oak tree, Olivia and Mr. Harold find comfort in each other's company, proving that age is just a number.

One day, as they were walking through the park, Mr. Harold stopped to admire a group of youngsters engrossed in their smartphones. Intrigued, he turned to Olivia and asked, "What is this fascination with small screens? Back in my day, we found joy in simpler things."

Olivia, always ready with a smile, replied:

Technology has its benefits, but the magic lies in finding the balance. Let me show you how these screens can connect us to the world in beautiful ways.

With Olivia's patient guidance, Mr. Harold tentatively entered the digital realm. Together they explored the wonders of video calls, virtual museums and online storytelling platforms. As Mr. Harold marveled at the possibilities, he realized that embracing change does not mean abandoning the past; it meant the enrichment of the present.

Their intergenerational bond became a beacon of inspiration for Eldridge. The community, initially skeptical of the unlikely friendship, came to see the value in bridging the generation gap. Soon, a program was started at the community center to encourage more interaction between young people and the elderly.

The story of Olivia and Mr. Harold touched the hearts of many and Eldridge Park was transformed into a symbol of unity. Young people have learned valuable lessons from their elders and gained insights that textbooks cannot provide. In return, the elderly felt rejuvenated by the contagious energy of youth.

As the seasons changed, so did the Eldridge dynamic. A city that once seemed divided by age now embraces the beauty of diversity. Eldridge became a canvas where stories of the past blended seamlessly with dreams of the future.

One crisp fall day, under the same oak tree where their journey began, Olivia and Mr. Harold pondered the impact of their friendship. Olivia expressed gratitude for the wisdom Mr. Harold shared while he marveled at the resilience and creativity of the younger generation.

As the sun sank below the horizon, casting a warm glow over the city, Olivia said, "Mr. Harold, our friendship proves that age is only a chapter in the book of life. What matters most is the story we create together."

Mr. Harold nodded with a twinkle in his eye. "Indeed, my dear. The real magic lies in the chapters we share, each generation adding a unique hue to the canvas of time."

And so, in Eldridge's heart, the intergenerational story of Olivia and Mr. Harold became a living testament to the beauty that unfolds when young and old walk hand in hand, weaving a story that transcends age and stands as a testament to the timeless power of connection.

Intergenerational relationships weave the intricate fabric of our society, connecting individuals across age gaps and fostering a mosaic of shared experiences, wisdom and understanding. In a world where the pace of change seems to accelerate every day, these connections become bridges that bridge generational gaps and offer a unique blend of perspectives that enrich the lives of young and old alike. As we embark on a journey to explore the dynamics of intergenerational relationships, we unravel the threads that connect grandparents and grandchildren, mentors and protégés, and the myriad connections that transcend time to create a vibrant mosaic of shared history and collective growth.

At the heart of intergenerational relationships lies the essence of human connection – a timeless dance between past and present, tradition and innovation. Grandparents, with their wrinkled hands and stories from a bygone era, become living vessels of history, passing on not just stories but a deep sense of identity rooted in the rich soil of heritage. At the same time, grandchildren bring a new perspective and navigate a world shaped by ever-evolving technology and social norms. This intersection of ages creates a harmonious blend where the old find rejuvenation through the lens of youth and the young gain a compass to navigate life's complexities from the wisdom of their elders.

In addition to family ties, intergenerational relationships take many forms, from mentoring programs in educational institutions to collaborative efforts in the workplace. The transfer of knowledge and skills from one generation to the next becomes a vital currency that fosters an environment where experience meets innovation. Seasoned professionals guide their younger counterparts and offer insights gained from years of trials and triumphs. In return, the younger generation injects vitality into established systems, challenges norms and drives progress. This symbiotic relationship drives society forward and ensures continuity of growth and adaptation.

But the beauty of intergenerational relationships goes beyond the exchange of knowledge—it permeates the emotional landscape. Laughter shared between grandparents and grandchildren echoes through the corridors of time, bridging the gaps with the universal language of joy. Similarly, mentoring relationships often transcend the professional sphere and develop into bonds based on mutual respect and genuine care. These connections serve as emotional anchors, provide support during life's storms, and celebrate victories, big and small. In a world where isolation can often be pervasive, intergenerational relationships emerge as beacons of connection that weave a safety net that transcends generational isolation.

However, orientation in the field of intergenerational relations is not without problems. A generation gap, often characterized by differences in values, communication styles and worldviews, can sow the seeds of misunderstanding. Bridging these gaps requires a delicate dance of empathy and openness, where each side tries to understand the other's point of view without judgment. It is in this dance that growth occurs as both generations learn to navigate the ever-changing environment of social norms and expectations.

As societies evolve, so do the dynamics of intergenerational relationships. The advent of the digital age has ushered in a new era of connectivity, allowing grandparents to share life's moments with their grandchildren across vast distances through video calls and social media. Similarly, mentoring has transcended physical proximity, virtual connection breaks down geographical barriers and fosters collaboration on a global scale. While the means of connection have evolved, the essence remains unchanged - the interweaving of lives across the tapestry of time.

It can be said that intergenerational relationships stand as pillars of strength in the edifice of human connection. They transcend age and create a story that speaks to the enduring power of shared experiences and mutual growth. As we navigate the currents of change, these relationships become compass points that guide us through the complexities of life with the wisdom of the past and the vigor of the present. In celebrating the diverse forms of these connections, we recognize their essential role in shaping not only individuals, but the very fabric of our interconnected society.

Chapter 1 Bridging the Gap: Understanding Intergenerational Dynamics

Intergenerational dynamics play a vital role in shaping our society, influencing everything from cultural norms to family structures. In today's world, where different generations exist side by side, understanding and orientation in intergenerational relationships is increasingly important. This article delves into the complexities of intergenerational dynamics, examines the factors that contribute to generational differences, and offers insight into how to bridge these differences.

Defining intergenerational dynamics:
Intergenerational dynamics refer to the interactions, conflicts, and shared experiences between individuals of different age groups within a society. These dynamics are shaped by a variety of factors,

including cultural changes, technological advances, economic shifts, and evolving societal expectations. Understanding these dynamics is essential to fostering healthy relationships and fostering social cohesion across generations.

Factors contributing to generational differences:
1. Technology division:

Rapid technological advancements have led to significant digital transformation and created a technology gap between generations. Younger generations, often referred to as digital natives, navigate the digital landscape effortlessly, while older generations may struggle to adapt. This division can lead to miscommunication and feelings of alienation.

2. Cultural Evolution:

Cultural norms and values evolve over time, contributing to generational differences. A younger generation may embrace progressive ideas and challenge traditional beliefs, causing tension with older generations who may hold more conservative views. Understanding and respecting these cultural shifts is essential to foster mutual understanding.

3. Economic differences:

Economic conditions and opportunities differ between generations. Older generations may have experienced a different economic reality, leading to different perspectives on financial stability, career choices, and overall life expectancy. Recognizing these differences is essential to resolving potential misunderstandings.

Navigating intergenerational relationships:
1. Open communication:

Effective communication is the key to bridging generational differences. Encouraging open dialogue allows individuals of different age groups to express their perspective, share experiences, and gain mutual insight into others' worldviews. Active listening is equally important for promoting understanding.

2. Cultural Exchange:

Promoting cultural exchange activities can help break down stereotypes and build empathy. Encouraging older generations to participate in activities popular with younger generations and vice versa can create shared experiences that transcend age differences.

3. Education and Awareness:

Educational programs aimed at promoting intergenerational understanding can be valuable. Schools, community centers and workplaces can implement initiatives that highlight the contributions of different generations, dispel stereotypes and highlight the shared values that unite us all.

Benefits of strong intergenerational relationships:
1. Transferring Wisdom:

Older generations have a wealth of experience and wisdom that can be invaluable to younger individuals. Establishing strong intergenerational ties enables the transfer of knowledge and life lessons, which contributes to personal growth and development.

2. Social Cohesion:

Healthy intergenerational relationships contribute to a sense of community and social cohesion. When individuals of different ages work together and support each other, it promotes a more open and harmonious society.

3. Innovation and Adaptability:

Combining the perspectives and skills of different generations can drive innovation. Younger individuals bring new ideas and technological knowledge, while older generations offer experience and historical context that can lead to informed decision-making.

Understanding intergenerational dynamics is key to building harmonious relationships across age groups. By acknowledging and addressing factors contributing to generational differences, society can create an environment that fosters mutual respect, collaboration and shared growth. Bridging the gap requires a commitment to open communication, cultural exchange and ongoing education to ensure a more connected and resilient society for future generations.

1.1 Exploring the foundations of intergenerational relationships

Intergenerational relationships, those that connect individuals from different age groups, play a key role in shaping societies and reinforcing a sense of continuity. These connections form the basis of social structures, influencing values, traditions and perspectives across generations. Understanding the foundations of intergenerational relationships involves delving into the dynamics that shape these connections, exploring their meaning, and recognizing the impact they have on individuals and communities.

One of the key aspects of intergenerational relationships is the passing on of values and traditions. Older generations often serve as custodians of cultural heritage, passing on beliefs, rituals, and customs to younger members. This transfer of knowledge not only preserves the community's identity, but also provides a sense of belonging and continuity. For example, grandparents can share stories from their past, impart wisdom, and instill a strong cultural identity in their grandchildren.

Furthermore, intergenerational relationships contribute to the development of empathy and understanding. When individuals from different age groups interact, they gain mutual insight into their experiences, challenges, and perspectives. This exchange fosters mutual respect and a deeper appreciation of different life paths. For example, a teenager can learn about historical events from a grandparent, gain a broader understanding of the world, and develop empathy for the struggles faced by previous generations.

Another critical aspect is the role of intergenerational relationships in shaping social norms and values. As older generations pass on their wisdom, younger individuals learn not only about cultural traditions, but also about ethical principles and moral values. This transmission helps maintain a sense of moral compass in communities and promotes social cohesion. For example, family gatherings provide opportunities for intergenerational dialogue where values such as respect, integrity and compassion are reinforced and shared.

Intergenerational relationships also play a vital role in the emotional well-being of individuals. The support and guidance provided by older family members contributes to a sense of security and stability. Research shows that, for example, strong bonds with grandparents can have a positive effect on children's emotional development and provide them with a wider support network beyond their immediate family. The emotional bonds created in intergenerational relationships create a sense of belonging and reduce feelings of isolation.

In addition, these relationships can bridge generational gaps, foster collaboration and innovation. In a rapidly changing world, older individuals bring valuable experience and perspective, while younger generations bring new ideas and technological knowledge. By working together, different age groups can tap into each generation's strengths, leading to creative solutions and progress. Collaborative initiatives that involve different age groups often produce more comprehensive and sustainable results.

However, there are also challenges in intergenerational relationships, primarily due to differences in communication styles, values, and lifestyles. Overcoming these differences requires an open mind and effective communication. Creating spaces for intergenerational dialogue where individuals feel comfortable expressing their opinions can facilitate understanding and bridge generational differences. Recognizing the importance of adapting to changing social norms and embracing diversity in age groups is essential to the success of intergenerational relationships.

Examining the foundations of intergenerational relationships reveals their profound impact on individuals and societies. From passing on cultural heritage to developing empathy and shaping social norms, these connections contribute to the fabric of communities. Recognizing and fostering positive intergenerational relationships is critical to creating resilient, inclusive societies that benefit from the strengths and perspectives of each generation.

1.2 Identifying key factors that shape generational perspectives

Understanding the dynamics of intergenerational relationships requires a close examination of the key factors that shape generational perspectives. These factors contribute to the unique ways in which individuals of different age groups perceive the world, interact with each other, and navigate the complexities of their shared experiences. In this survey, we delve into several critical elements that play a key role in shaping generational perspectives in the context of intergenerational relationships.

1. Historical events and cultural shifts:
One of the primary determinants of generational perspectives is the impact of historical events and cultural shifts. Each generation is deeply influenced by significant events that occurred during their formative years. For example, individuals who grew up in times of economic prosperity may approach life with a sense of optimism and self-confidence, while those who have experienced periods of

economic decline may exhibit more cautious and pragmatic attitudes. In addition, cultural movements, technological advances, and political shifts contribute to the formation of distinct generational identities.

2. Technological Advancement:

The rapid development of technology is a defining feature of modern times and significantly shapes the perspectives of different generations. Older generations may view technological advances with a degree of skepticism, while younger generations readily accept and integrate new technologies into their lives. The digital divide therefore becomes a crucial factor influencing how individuals of different age groups communicate, access information and interpret the world around them.

3. Economic landscape:

The economic conditions prevailing during a generation's adolescence play a key role in shaping their perspective on financial stability, work and success. Generations that have experienced economic prosperity may prioritize career advancement and material success, while those that have endured economic hardship may value stability, frugality, and long-term planning. These different priorities can lead to misunderstandings and conflicts in intergenerational relationships.

4. Social and political movements:
Generational perspectives are intricately tied to the social and political movements that shaped their era. Individuals who have witnessed or participated in transformative movements such as civil rights, feminism, or environmental activism can carry these values into their intergenerational interactions. Understanding the social and political context in which each generation grew up is essential to fostering empathy and bridging ideological divides within family and community relationships.

5. Education and Cultural Exposure:
Educational experiences and cultural exposure contribute significantly to generational perspectives. The type of education individuals receive, the cultural diversity they encounter, and the values

instilled during their formative years all influence how they perceive the world and how they treat others. Intergenerational relationships can be enriched by recognizing and appreciating the diversity of educational and cultural backgrounds that each generation brings to the table.

6. Change in family structures:

The structure of families has evolved over time and influenced generational views of relationships, gender roles, and family dynamics. Traditional family structures, characterized by clear hierarchies and defined roles, have given way to more fluid and egalitarian models. Understanding these shifts is critical to navigating intergenerational relationships, as expectations and norms can differ significantly between generations.

7. Communication styles:

Generations often develop different communication styles influenced by the prevailing modes of communication during their formation. Older generations may value face-to-face communication and traditional etiquette, while younger generations may rely heavily on digital communication platforms and prefer informal and quick exchanges. Recognizing and accommodating these differences is necessary to promote effective communication and mutual understanding.

Identifying the key factors that shape generational perspectives is essential to fostering healthy and constructive intergenerational relationships. By acknowledging the influence of historical events, technological advances, the economic landscape, social and political movements, education, changing family structures, and communication styles, individuals can bridge the generation gap and build connections based on understanding and empathy. Embracing the diversity of generational perspectives contributes to a more harmonious coexistence, allowing each generation to learn from the other and navigate the ever-changing landscape of human experience together.

Chapter 2 Communication Across Ages: Navigating Generational Differences

In a rapidly changing world, intergenerational relationships are increasingly prevalent, bringing together individuals from different age groups with different perspectives, values and communication styles. Effective communication across generations is essential to promote understanding, cooperation and harmony in various social and professional settings. This contextual examination delves into the dynamics of communication across the ages and illuminates the challenges and opportunities presented by generational differences in the context of intergenerational relationships.

Understanding Generational Differences:
Generational differences involve a wide range of factors, including communication preferences, work

styles and cultural influences. Key generations often referenced in discussions of this topic include the Silent Generation, Baby Boomers, Generation X, Millennials, and Generation Z. Each cohort has been shaped by unique historical events, technological advances, and societal shifts that have contributed to distinct worldviews that affect the message.

1. The Silent Generation and Baby Boomers:
Members of the Silent Generation and Baby Boomers often value face-to-face communication and traditional workplace hierarchy. With experiences rooted in pre-digital times, they may prefer formal modes of communication and hierarchical structures. Understanding their appreciation of loyalty and respect can strengthen intergenerational interactions.

2. Generation X:
Positioned between Baby Boomers and Millennials, Generation X tends to value independence and work-life balance. Their communication style is often pragmatic and straightforward. Recognizing

their skepticism towards authority and preference for autonomy can promote more effective communication in personal and professional relationships.

3. Millennials:

Having witnessed the rise of the internet, millennials are characterized by a tech-savvy mindset and a desire for meaningful connections. They often favor digital communication channels and a collaborative, inclusive environment. Recognizing their emphasis on purpose-driven work and constant connectivity is essential to navigating relationships with this generation.

4. Generation Z:

The youngest generation, Generation Z, grew up in a hyper-connected, digitized world. They are known for their entrepreneurial spirit, diversity awareness and reliance on social media to communicate. Being aware of their fluid approach to work and life, as well as their preference for visual communication, is essential to fostering effective relationships.

Challenges in communication across the ages:

Despite the richness that different generational perspectives bring, problems can arise in communication due to different communication styles, technological knowledge and different expectations. Stereotyping and misinterpretation of intentions based on generational assumptions can hinder cooperation and create unnecessary conflicts.

1. Communication styles:

Different communication styles can lead to misunderstandings. For example, younger generations accustomed to fast, informal digital communication may find the formal communication styles of older generations slow and cumbersome. Bridging this gap requires a willingness to adapt communication strategies to suit the preferences of different age groups.

2. Technological capability:

The digital divide between generations can present barriers to communication. While younger generations can navigate the latest technology effortlessly, older generations may struggle to keep up. Promoting intergenerational learning opportunities and providing technological literacy support can alleviate this problem.

3. Workplace Expectations:
Generational differences in workplace expectations can create tension. For example, Baby Boomers may prefer loyalty to work, while Millennials may seek purpose-driven work and career flexibility. Organizations must strive to create an inclusive environment that accommodates diverse expectations and fosters a sense of belonging for individuals of all ages.

Opportunities for effective communication:
Managing generational differences in communication within intergenerational relationships presents numerous opportunities for growth, collaboration, and the exchange of valuable insights. By recognizing and embracing diversity, individuals and organizations can leverage the strengths inherent in multigenerational teams.

1. Knowledge Exchange:

Each generation brings rich experience and knowledge. Facilitating knowledge exchange programs where individuals from different age groups can share their expertise fosters a culture of continuous learning and mutual respect. This approach not only enhances individual development, but also contributes to the collective wisdom of the group.

2. Mentorship Programs:

Establishing mentoring programs that bring together individuals from different generations fosters meaningful connections. Younger generations can benefit from the wisdom and guidance of older mentors, while older generations gain new perspectives and insights from their mentees. This mutual relationship fosters a supportive environment that transcends generational boundaries.

3. Flexible communication strategy:

Organizations and individuals are aware of the diversity of communication preferences and can adopt flexible communication strategies. This can include a combination of traditional face-to-face communication, digital channels and customized approaches based on specific audience needs. Adapting communication styles to generational differences increases overall effectiveness.

We can say that effective communication across the ages is key to the success of intergenerational relationships. By understanding and appreciating the unique perspectives, values, and communication styles of different generations, individuals and organizations can foster an environment that fosters collaboration, innovation, and personal growth. Embracing the opportunities offered by generational diversity and addressing challenges through open dialogue and adaptability contribute to creating inclusive spaces where individuals of all ages can thrive.

2.1 Strategies for effective communication between generations

Effective intergenerational communication is essential to fostering positive intergenerational relationships. At a time when different age groups coexist in different settings such as workplaces, families and communities, understanding and implementing strategies for successful communication can bridge generational gaps and promote harmony. This contextual content will explore key strategies for effective intergenerational communication and emphasize the importance of mutual respect, empathy, and openness.

1. Understanding Generational Differences:

In order to communicate effectively across generations, it is essential to recognize and appreciate the distinct characteristics and values that each generation brings. Generational differences in communication styles, work ethics and perspectives can lead to misunderstandings if not acknowledged. By understanding these differences, individuals can adjust their communication approach to create a more inclusive and harmonious environment.

2. Active listening:

Active listening is an essential component of effective communication. Generations can perceive and process information differently, so active listening is key to understanding different perspectives. Encouraging open dialogue and providing undivided attention during conversations can improve understanding and foster a sense of appreciation between individuals of different age groups.

3. Versatile technology:

In today's digital age, technology plays a significant role in communication. Younger generations may be more accustomed to using digital platforms, while older generations may prefer traditional forms of communication. Finding common ground by embracing technology where appropriate and respecting traditional communication methods can create a balanced approach that accommodates different preferences.

4. Establishing common goals:

Identifying shared goals helps unite generations towards a common purpose. Whether in a professional or family setting, aligning goals creates a sense of unity and fosters cooperation. Clearly articulating these shared goals fosters a sense of purpose and fosters a positive atmosphere for effective communication.

5. Building Empathy:

Developing empathy is essential to understanding the experiences and perspectives of different generations. Each generation faced unique challenges and societal shifts that contributed to different worldviews. Empathy allows individuals to appreciate these differences and build connections based on shared emotions and experiences.

6. Mentoring programs:

Establishing mentoring programs can facilitate the exchange of knowledge and skills between generations. Younger individuals can benefit from the wisdom and experience of older mentors, while older individuals can gain new perspectives and insights from their mentees. This mutual exchange not only strengthens communication, but also strengthens intergenerational relationships.

7. Flexibility in communication styles:

It is essential to realize that communication styles differ between generations. While younger generations may prefer brief and direct communication, older generations may appreciate more formal and detailed conversations. Adapting communication styles based on the preferences of the individuals involved contributes to a more effective exchange of ideas.

8. Support for intergenerational cooperation:

Actively encouraging collaboration between different age groups fosters a sense of unity and shared responsibility. Whether in the workplace or within communities, intergenerational collaboration can lead to innovative solutions and a more inclusive environment. Creating opportunities for joint projects or initiatives promotes communication and collaboration.

9. Providing generational sensitivity training:

Organizations and institutions can play a key role in promoting effective communication by offering generational sensitivity training programs. These programs can educate individuals about the characteristics, values and communication preferences of different generations and promote a more informed and inclusive environment.

10. Celebrating Diversity:

Embracing generational diversity involves celebrating the strengths each generation brings to the table. Acknowledging and valuing the unique perspectives, skills and experiences of individuals from different age groups contributes to a culture of recognition and respect.

Effective intergenerational communication is a dynamic process that requires understanding, adaptability, and commitment to building meaningful connections. By implementing these strategies, individuals and organizations can create an environment where different age groups work harmoniously together and contribute to the common success and well-being of all parties involved.

2.2 Overcoming challenges and fostering mutual understanding

Intergenerational relationships, marked by differences in age, experience, and perspective, often present unique challenges. Overcoming these barriers requires a concerted effort to promote mutual understanding and bridge the generation gap. In a world where technology, social norms and values are rapidly evolving, the dynamics between different age groups can be complex. This essay delves into the challenges facing intergenerational relationships and explores strategies to overcome them, emphasizing the importance of open communication, empathy, and shared experiences. One of the main challenges in intergenerational relationships are differences in life experiences and perspectives. Older generations may have grown up in a completely different socio-political environment and faced challenges and opportunities different from those encountered by younger generations. This division can result in a lack of understanding and appreciation for each other's backgrounds, leading to miscommunication and potential conflict.

Promoting mutual understanding is paramount to solving this problem. Fostering open and honest communication is an essential first step. Both parties must be willing to share their experiences, perspectives, and values without judgment. This exchange can provide valuable insights into the factors that shaped each generation and lay the groundwork for empathy and connection.

Furthermore, it is essential to acknowledge differences without assigning blame. Instead of seeing differences as obstacles, they can be seen as opportunities to learn and grow. Older generations can offer wisdom and historical context, while younger generations bring fresh perspectives and innovative ideas. Recognizing the value in these differences creates a more inclusive environment where both sides feel heard and respected.

Another significant challenge is the technological advancement that has changed the way people interact and communicate. Older generations may feel overwhelmed or left behind by the rapid pace of technological change, leading to a communication gap with their younger counterparts. Bridging this gap requires patience, education, and a willingness to embrace new ways of connecting.

Younger individuals can play a key role in facilitating technological literacy among older generations. Offering guidance in the use of digital platforms, social media and other modern communication tools can empower older individuals and strengthen their connection with the younger generation. At the same time, older individuals can share their rich life experiences and create an environment of mutual learning.

In addition, intergenerational relationships often face challenges related to differing cultural norms and societal expectations. Each generation is shaped by the cultural context in which it grew up and influences its values, beliefs and behavior. Navigating these differences requires a commitment to understanding and respecting different perspectives.

Promoting cultural sensitivity involves actively engaging in conversations about traditions, values, and societal expectations. This exchange allows each generation to gain insight into the worldview of the others and fosters a sense of cultural appreciation. Celebrating shared values and finding common ground can strengthen the bond between generations and create a more harmonious relationship.

In addition to communication and understanding, shared experiences play a vital role in building stronger intergenerational relationships. Activities that bridge generational gaps, such as family reunions, community events, or joint projects, provide opportunities for meaningful interaction. These shared experiences create lasting memories and a sense of unity, transcending age-related barriers.

To overcome problems in intergenerational relationships, it is necessary to cultivate a mindset of continuous learning and adaptation. Both older and younger individuals must be open to accepting new perspectives, questioning their assumptions and evolving with the changing times. This willingness to adapt promotes resilience and ensures that intergenerational relationships remain dynamic and fulfilling.

Overcoming challenges in intergenerational relationships requires a multifaceted approach that prioritizes communication, empathy, and shared experiences. By fostering mutual understanding, acknowledging differences without judgment, embracing technological literacy, fostering cultural sensitivity, and engaging in joint activities, individuals can bridge the generation gap and build stronger connections across age groups. In a world characterized by diversity and change, cultivating meaningful intergenerational relationships is not only beneficial for personal growth, but also essential to creating a more inclusive and harmonious society .

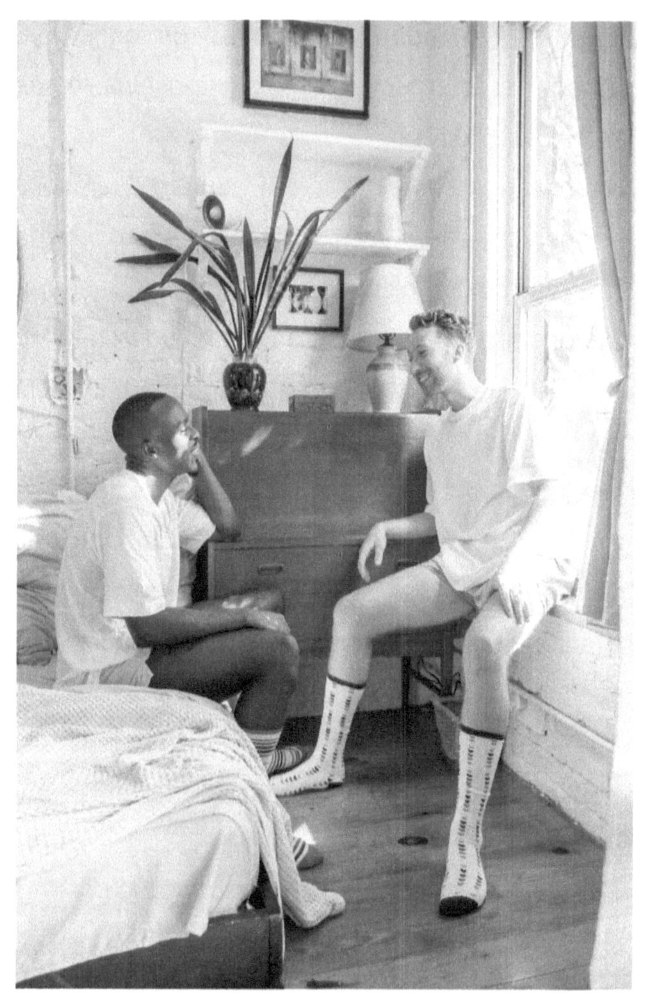

Chapter 3 Passing Down Wisdom: The Art of Intergenerational Mentoring

Intergenerational mentoring is a timeless practice that involves the transfer of knowledge, skills and life lessons from one generation to the next. It is a deep form of connection that fosters understanding, empathy and a sense of continuity across age groups. In this survey, we will delve into the importance of intergenerational mentoring and its impact on relationships between different generations.

Understanding Intergenerational Mentoring:

Intergenerational mentoring is not a universal concept; it includes a spectrum of interactions between individuals of different age groups. It involves sharing experiences, insights and practical wisdom, creating a bridge that bridges the gaps between generations. This dynamic exchange goes beyond the mere transfer of information; it involves a reciprocal process where both mentor and mentee contribute to the growth and enrichment of their lives.

The role of wisdom in intergenerational mentoring:

Wisdom, often accumulated through a lifetime of experience, is a central component of intergenerational mentoring. A mentor who has a wealth of knowledge imparts valuable lessons that go beyond textbooks or formal education. These teachings touch on the nuances of life and provide the mentee with a compass to navigate the complexities of their own path.

Wisdom in this context is not just knowing facts or having information; it's about understanding the deeper currents of life, being able to make sound judgments, and having a perspective that goes beyond the immediate present. Through intergenerational mentoring, this wisdom becomes a living legacy, passed down from generation to generation.

Building bridges across generations:

Intergenerational mentoring serves as a powerful bridge connecting individuals who might otherwise remain isolated within their respective age groups. It promotes a sense of continuity, breaks down stereotypes and preconceived notions about different generations. As the older generation passes on their wisdom, the younger generation brings new perspectives, innovative ideas and keen awareness of contemporary challenges.
This exchange benefits both parties and creates a harmonious synergy where the strengths of one generation complement the vitality of the other. The mentor learns to adapt to changing times, to remain relevant and engaged, while the mentee gains a historical perspective, appreciating the roots from which he grew.

Caring for emotional intelligence:

In addition to the transfer of knowledge, intergenerational mentoring plays a key role in the development of emotional intelligence. Drawing on their life experiences, the mentor offers insight into managing emotions, resolving conflict and building resilience. These lessons, often learned through trial and error, become invaluable tools for mentees in navigating the complex landscape of human relationships.

Additionally, the emotional connection created through mentoring creates a support system that extends beyond family ties. It creates a sense of belonging and security and supports the emotional well-being of both mentor and mentee. In a rapidly changing world where the pace of life can be overwhelming, this emotional anchor becomes a stabilizing force.

Breaking down stereotypes and promoting mutual respec:t

Stereotypes and misconceptions about different generations prevail in society. Intergenerational mentoring challenges these stereotypes by providing opportunities for individuals to interact on a personal level. When mentor and mentee engage in open dialogue, they discover shared values, aspirations, and challenges, disrupting preconceived notions that may have been based on generational misunderstandings.

This process of mutual discovery fosters respect and appreciation for the unique strengths each generation brings to the table. The mentor learns to appreciate the energy and innovation of the younger generation, while the mentee gains an understanding of the wisdom that comes with experience. This mutual respect forms the basis for a more harmonious and connected society.

Solving the digital generation gap:

In the digital age, where technology is developing at an unprecedented pace, a significant generation gap has emerged. Intergenerational mentoring is becoming a vital tool for bridging this gap as older generations share their insights into a world that has rapidly changed over the years. The mentor provides guidance on navigating the digital environment while the mentee introduces the mentor to the latest technological advances.

This exchange not only facilitates technological literacy, but also creates a space for meaningful discussions about the societal impact of technology. Through intergenerational mentoring, both generations can work together to take advantage of technology and mitigate its potential disadvantages.

The reciprocal nature of intergenerational mentoring:

While the mentor imparts wisdom, the mentee brings new perspectives and a renewed sense of curiosity to the relationship. This reciprocity makes intergenerational mentoring a dynamic and evolving process. A mentor is not just a giver of knowledge; they are also receivers, gaining insight into the evolving dynamics of society, culture and aspirations of younger generations.

In turn, the mentee benefits not only from the mentor's wisdom, but also from his openness to new ideas and willingness to accept change. This mutual exchange creates a symbiotic relationship that transcends the traditional mentor-mentee dynamic and fosters a sense of partnership and shared growth.

Overcoming challenges in intergenerational mentoring:

While the benefits of intergenerational mentoring are profound, it is essential to recognize and address potential challenges. Poor communication, generational biases, and resistance to change can be obstacles to the smooth flow of wisdom between generations. Creating a supportive and open environment where both mentor and mentee feel heard and respected is critical to overcoming these challenges.

Creating clear communication channels, setting realistic expectations, and fostering a culture of openness can contribute to the success of intergenerational mentoring relationships. In addition, realizing that learning is a two-way street promotes a mindset of constant growth and adaptability.

Intergenerational mentoring is a rich tapestry woven with threads of wisdom, empathy and mutual respect. It is a testament to the enduring power of human connection at different stages of life. As society continues to evolve, the art of imparting wisdom becomes not only a tradition, but a necessity for navigating the complexities of an ever-changing world

When supporting the intergenerational.

3.1 Examining mentorship as a powerful tool for knowledge transfer

Mentoring, a dynamic process of knowledge transfer and personal development, is proving to be a powerful tool in the complex tapestry of intergenerational relationships. As societies evolve, the exchange of wisdom between generations becomes increasingly important, fostering continuous learning that transcends age and experience. This essay delves into the multifaceted realm of mentoring, dissecting its meaning in the context of intergenerational relationships and elucidating how it serves as a conduit for the seamless transfer of knowledge across eras.

At its core, mentoring encapsulates a mutual relationship where an experienced individual guides and supports a less experienced counterpart, supporting their personal and professional growth. In the context of intergenerational dynamics, this mentor-mentee relationship goes beyond mere guardianship; it becomes a bridge connecting different periods of life, each characterized by unique challenges, perspectives and insights. The interplay between experienced mentors and eager mentees creates an invaluable channel for the transmission of accumulated knowledge, skills and cultural nuances that might otherwise dissipate across generations.

One of the fundamental aspects of mentoring in intergenerational relationships lies in its ability to counteract the potential erosion of wisdom that can occur when a societal paradigm changes. The rapid pace of technological progress and evolving social norms often leaves a generation gap where the experiences and lessons of the past are at risk of being overlooked or undervalued. Mentorship becomes an insurance policy against this information depletion, offering a means of preserving and passing on time-tested wisdom to the next generation.

In addition, mentorship serves as a catalyst for innovation and adaptability in the face of changing landscapes. Intergenerational mentoring combines the insight of established mentors who have weathered the storms of years past with the fresh perspectives and untapped potential of mentees navigating the current environment. This combination of experience and youthful exuberance creates an environment conducive to creative problem solving and the cultivation of forward-thinking ideas.

The mentorship paradigm also plays a key role in addressing the psychological and emotional dimensions of intergenerational relationships. As individuals navigate the complexities of life, having a mentor from another generation provides a unique perspective. Mentors can offer insights derived from their own life experiences, helping mentees navigate challenges, make informed decisions, and develop resilience in the face of adversity. This emotional support is especially important in a world where social dynamics and individual aspirations are constantly evolving.

In addition, the mentoring dynamic within intergenerational relationships contributes to building social cohesion and understanding. By fostering meaningful connections between individuals of different ages, mentoring fosters empathy and a shared sense of purpose. Mentors, drawing on their experiences, can bridge generational gaps by facilitating open dialogue and mutual understanding. This not only enriches the mentee's personal development, but also cultivates a sense of interconnectedness that transcends individual relationships and has a positive impact on the wider community.

Practically speaking, the implementation of effective intergenerational mentoring programs can occur in a variety of contexts, including educational institutions, workplaces, and community settings. Educational institutions can harness the power of mentorship to create a holistic learning environment where academic knowledge is blended with real-world insights. Workplaces can implement mentorship programs to facilitate the seamless integration of new talent and ensure the transfer of institutional knowledge that goes beyond procedural manuals. Community mentoring initiatives can bridge gaps between different age groups and foster a sense of community and collective responsibility.

However, despite its myriad benefits, the effectiveness of intergenerational mentoring depends on several critical factors. One key aspect is cultivating a supportive mentoring culture that values the exchange of ideas across generations. This includes breaking down age-related stereotypes and recognizing the unique strengths each generation brings to the table. Creating mentoring opportunities that are inclusive, flexible and tailored to the needs of both mentors and mentees is paramount to fostering a sustainable and mutually beneficial mentoring ecosystem.

In addition, recognizing the evolving nature of knowledge is essential in designing mentoring programs that remain relevant across generations. The mentoring environment must adapt to the changing dynamics of a globalized, technology-driven world and ensure that mentees are equipped not only with traditional wisdom, but also with the skills and adaptability needed to thrive in contemporary contexts.

Examining mentoring as a powerful tool for knowledge transfer within intergenerational relationships reveals a number of benefits that go beyond individual growth. As the interplay between experienced mentors and eager mentees weaves together the threads of the past, present and future, mentorship proves to be a foundational pillar for the continuity of wisdom, innovation and emotional support across generations. To reach its full potential, society must foster a culture that values and nurtures intergenerational mentorship and recognizes it as a cornerstone for building resilient, connected communities ready for continuous growth and adaptation.

3.2 Case studies on successful intergenerational mentorship

Intergenerational mentoring has proven to be a powerful tool for fostering meaningful connections across different age groups. Successful case studies in this area show the transformative impact such relationships can have on individuals and communities. By examining cases where intergenerational mentoring has been successful, we gain valuable insights into the dynamics that contribute to its success and its broader implications for intergenerational relationships.

One notable case study is the "Generations Connect" program initiated by a local community organization. This program paired experienced professionals, mostly from the baby boom generation, with young professionals just entering the workforce. Structured mentoring sessions provided a platform to exchange knowledge, skills and perspectives. Older mentors offered insights gained through years of experience, while younger mentees brought new ideas and technological knowledge.

The success of this program was attributed to its intentional focus on creating an environment of mutual learning. Both mentors and mentees were encouraged to openly share their experiences, challenges and aspirations. This two-way exchange not only improved the skills of the mentees but also allowed the mentors to keep abreast of current trends and technologies. The result was a symbiotic relationship that transcended generational gaps.

Similarly, in a corporate environment, a multinational company introduced an intergenerational mentoring initiative to bridge the gap between experienced managers and younger employees. Through carefully selected mentoring pairs, the company has focused on facilitating knowledge transfer, leadership development and a sense of unity among its diverse workforce.

One of the key elements contributing to the success of this program was the emphasis on personalized mentoring plans. Rather than adopting a one-size-fits-all approach, mentors and mentees jointly outline goals and expectations, ensuring that mentoring is tailored to each individual's specific needs and aspirations. This adaptation fostered a deeper connection and increased the relevance of mentoring in the professional development of the participants.

The impact of successful intergenerational mentoring goes beyond the individual level and affects organizational culture. In another case study within the education sector, a university implemented a mentoring program that pairs senior faculty members with junior faculty members. This initiative not only supported the career development of junior academics, but also contributed to greater collaboration and a supportive institutional culture.

The success of this program was attributed to its deliberate integration into the university's overall strategic plan. By linking intergenerational mentoring to broader institutional goals, the university ensured that mentoring was seen as a key part of professional development rather than an isolated initiative. This strategic integration led to a cultural shift where mentoring became embedded in the fabric of the academic community.

The case studies further highlight the importance of breaking down stereotypes and preconceived notions that can hinder effective intergenerational mentoring. In one particular case, a community organization sought to dispel misconceptions about the abilities and contributions of older adults. By actively involving older individuals as youth mentors in various educational and vocational programs, the organization has successfully tackled age-related stereotypes and fostered a sense of mutual respect and understanding.

The success of intergenerational mentoring in a variety of contexts underscores its potential to bridge generational gaps, promote learning, and create more inclusive and supportive communities. Key elements such as personalized mentoring plans, strategic integration into organizational goals, and challenging stereotypes contribute to the effectiveness of these programs. As we continue to explore and implement intergenerational mentoring initiatives, these case studies serve as valuable guides that offer insight into best practices and strategies for cultivating successful intergenerational relationships.

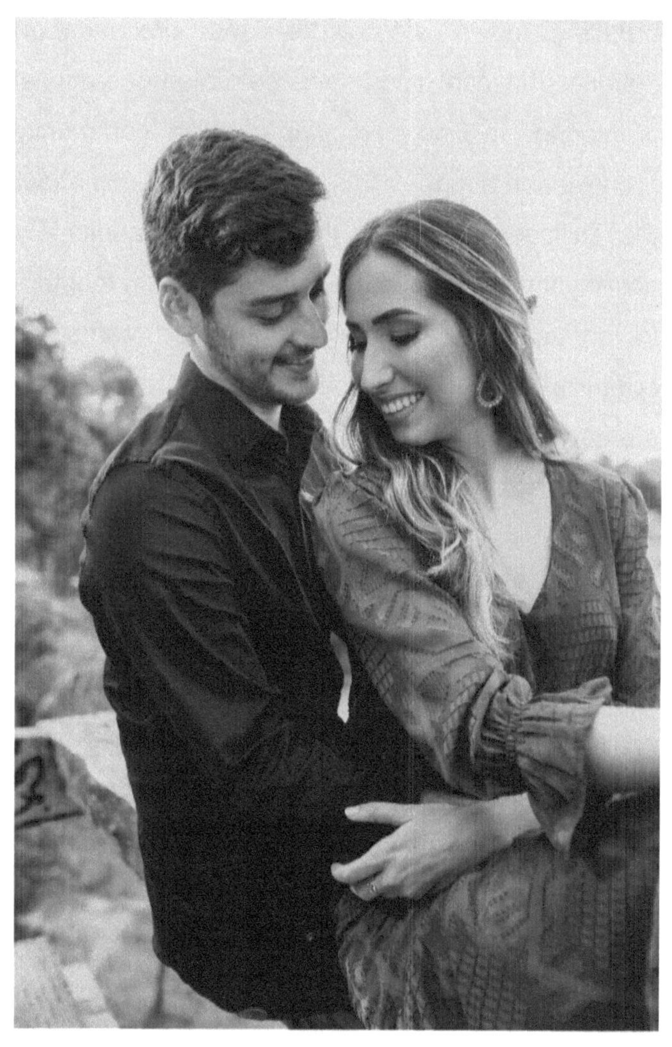

Chapter 4 The Future Together: Building Stronger Bonds Across Generations

Intergenerational relationships play a vital role in shaping the structure of societies. As we navigate the complexity of an ever-changing world, the connection between different age groups is increasingly important. "The Future Together" encapsulates the essence of strengthening stronger bonds across generations, presenting a harmonious coexistence that not only bridges the generation gap, but also drives society forward through shared wisdom, understanding and empathy.

In an age marked by rapid technological progress and an evolving cultural landscape, the intergenerational exchange of knowledge is paramount. The older generation brings rich experience, traditional values and historical perspectives to serve as a guiding force. At the same time, the younger generation contributes innovation, adaptability and a new perspective, paving the way forward. The synergy between these age groups forms the cornerstone of social progress.

One aspect of building stronger bonds across generations is recognizing and appreciating the unique strengths that each age group brings to the table. The older generation, often characterized by its wisdom and life experience, serves as a reservoir of knowledge. Their stories, anecdotes and historical contexts provide invaluable insights that serve as a compass for a younger generation navigating an increasingly complex world.

On the contrary, the younger generation, armed with technological skills and dynamic thinking, adds vitality to society. Their innovative thinking combined with a natural inclination to change propels the company forward. Embracing this interplay between experience and innovation is essential to building a future that is both rooted in tradition and adaptable to change.

Education is becoming a pivotal place for intergenerational cooperation. Traditional wisdom can be seamlessly integrated with modern pedagogical approaches to create a holistic learning environment. Mentoring programs, where experienced individuals guide and mentor the younger generation, offer a structured pathway for knowledge transfer. At the same time, the younger generation can provide insight into current challenges and foster a symbiotic relationship that enhances the overall educational experience.

Moreover, the workplace is a microcosm where intergenerational relationships significantly influence productivity and organizational culture. Companies that recognize and leverage the strengths of different age groups foster an environment of innovation and resilience. Mentoring programs, collaborative projects, and open communication channels create a workplace where experience and new perspectives blend, leading the organization to succeed.

The future of healthcare also benefits from intergenerational collaboration. As the population ages, the knowledge of older generations about health practices and preventive measures becomes invaluable. At the same time, younger generations are contributing to progress in the healthcare industry with their knowledge of cutting-edge medical technology and research. By fostering collaboration between different age groups, companies can address the challenges posed by an aging population while harnessing the potential for medical breakthroughs.

Intergenerational relationships are equally important in solving societal problems and promoting social cohesion. By promoting understanding and empathy between generations, companies can mitigate age-related stereotypes and prejudices. Encouraging dialogue and sharing experiences can break down barriers and foster a sense of community that transcends age. This interconnectedness is essential in addressing global challenges, from environmental sustainability to social justice, as it fosters collective responsibility that transcends generations.

However, building stronger ties across generations is not without challenges. Poor communication, stereotypes and resistance to change can create barriers between age groups. Bridging these gaps requires a concerted effort from both sides. Initiatives that facilitate intergenerational interactions, such as community events, workshops and collaborative projects, can provide platforms for mutual understanding.

Technology, often seen as a source of generational division, can also be used to strengthen intergenerational relationships. Virtual platforms can facilitate communication and collaboration, allowing individuals of different ages to connect and share experiences. In addition, educational resources and initiatives can be disseminated through digital channels, creating a more inclusive learning environment.

The Future Together: Building Stronger Bonds Across Generations" represents a society where the strengths of different age groups are used to progress together. By recognizing the value of intergenerational relationships in education, the workplace, healthcare and social cohesion, we are paving the way for a future rich in shared wisdom, innovation and empathy. The journey to building stronger bonds across generations is an ongoing process that requires active participation, an open mind, and a commitment to creating a world where each generation contributes to and benefits from the collective tapestry of human experience.

4.1 Creating inclusive environments for diverse age groups

Creating an inclusive environment for different age groups is crucial to fostering positive intergenerational relationships. In today's dynamic society, where people of different ages coexist in workplaces, communities and families, the need for inclusive spaces that celebrate and accommodate age differences has never been more critical.

First, an inclusive environment recognizes and values the unique perspectives, experiences, and contributions of individuals across age groups. This includes breaking down stereotypes and challenging age-related prejudices that may exist. By fostering an understanding and appreciation for the different experiences that come with different life stages, a more harmonious atmosphere and cooperation can be created.

In workplaces, adopting a multigenerational approach can lead to increased creativity and productivity. Younger individuals bring fresh perspectives and technological knowledge, while older employees bring valuable experience and wisdom. By recognizing and leveraging the strengths of each age group, organizations can cultivate a more innovative and dynamic workforce. Education is another area where inclusivity for different age groups is key. In educational settings, from schools to community programs, recognizing the unique learning styles and needs of different age groups can improve the overall learning experience. For example, incorporating mentoring programs that pair older students with younger ones creates opportunities for mutual learning and support.

Intergenerational relationships in families also benefit from an inclusive environment. Creating spaces where family members of all ages feel heard and valued fosters stronger bonds. Shared activities that target different age groups can become a bridge providing common ground for meaningful interactions. Grandparents, parents and children can engage in activities that satisfy their interests while finding shared experiences that strengthen their relationships.

Communities also play a vital role in promoting intergenerational inclusivity. Public spaces and events that cater to different age groups contribute to a sense of belonging for everyone. Parks with amenities for both children and seniors, community events that bring people of all ages together, and initiatives that encourage intergenerational collaboration all contribute to creating a more inclusive community.

Intergenerational inclusivity is not just about accommodating different age groups; it is an active search for ways to bridge generational gaps. This includes promoting communication and understanding between generations. Initiatives such as workshops, forums or community projects that involve individuals from different age groups can facilitate dialogue and help break down stereotypes.

In addition, the use of technology can be a powerful tool in creating intergenerational bonds. Older generations can benefit from the expertise of younger individuals in navigating digital platforms, while younger generations can learn from the experiences and stories shared by their elders. Technology can serve as a bridge, connecting people across generations and facilitating the exchange of knowledge and ideas.

In short, creating an inclusive environment for different age groups is a multifaceted effort that includes challenging stereotypes, recognizing the unique strengths of each generation, and actively promoting intergenerational relationships. Whether in workplaces, educational settings, families or communities, the benefits of promoting inclusivity are numerous. By embracing and celebrating the diversity that comes with different age groups, we can build stronger, more resilient and vibrant societies that honor the contributions of individuals at every stage of life.

4.2 Exploring the Impact of intergenerational relationships on society

Intergenerational relationships play a key role in shaping the structure of society, influencing cultural norms, values and the transmission of knowledge between generations. This dynamic interaction between individuals of different age groups fosters a sense of continuity and contributes to the social, emotional and intellectual development of communities. In this survey, we delve into the multifaceted impact of intergenerational relationships on society and examine how these connections affect social cohesion, individual well-being, and the transmission of wisdom.

The basis of intergenerational relations is the exchange of experiences and views. Older generations often serve as repositories of historical knowledge, traditional practices, and invaluable life lessons. When younger individuals meet their elders, they gain insight into the past and foster a deeper understanding of cultural roots and social development. This transmission of wisdom not only preserves heritage, but also provides a compass for navigating contemporary challenges.

In addition to the transfer of knowledge, intergenerational relationships also contribute significantly to emotional well-being. The companionship and support offered by these connections creates a sense of belonging and safety. For older individuals, interacting with younger generations can combat feelings of isolation and provide a renewed sense of purpose. Meanwhile, younger individuals benefit from the guidance and emotional stability that older mentors and role models can provide.

Intergenerational relationships also play a key role in shaping social attitudes and values. When different age groups interact, they bring different perspectives to the fore and promote tolerance and understanding. This intergenerational dialogue challenges stereotypes and helps break down age-related prejudices and promotes inclusiveness in society. The interplay between generations becomes a catalyst for cultural enrichment, leading to the creation of a more harmonious and integrated social landscape.

The impact of intergenerational relations also extends to the economic sphere. Older generations often have a wealth of professional experience and expertise. Through mentorship and knowledge transfer, they can guide younger individuals on their career path, accelerate skill development and foster innovation. This cross-generational collaboration contributes to a more robust and adaptable workforce and increases the overall economic resilience of society.

In the context of education, intergenerational relationships provide an additional pathway to learning. For example, grandparents can offer unique insights and support during a child's educational journey. Their involvement not only improves the child's academic results, but also strengthens family ties. In addition, older individuals benefit from the opportunity to remain mentally active and engaged through interactions with younger minds, creating a mutual and mutually beneficial learning environment.

Despite the many positive aspects of intergenerational relationships, there are also challenges. Generation gaps can lead to miscommunication and misunderstandings. Bridging these gaps requires open dialogue, empathy and a willingness to appreciate different perspectives. Additionally, societal changes such as mobility and evolving family structures can affect the frequency and nature of intergenerational interactions. Recognizing and addressing these challenges is essential to maintaining and enhancing the positive impact of intergenerational connections.

Examining the impact of intergenerational relationships on society reveals a complex web of influences that span cultural, emotional, economic, and educational dimensions. These relationships contribute to the richness and resilience of societies, fostering a sense of continuity, emotional well-being and cultural diversity. As we navigate the complexity of our ever-evolving world, recognizing and maintaining the importance of intergenerational connections remains critical to building stronger, more cohesive communities.

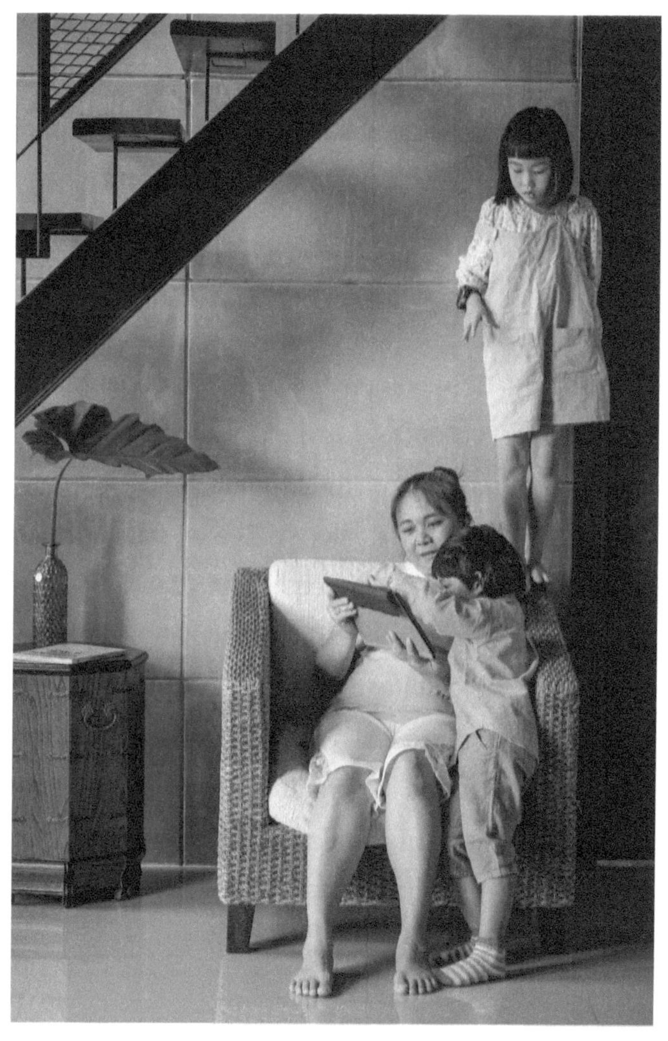

CONCLUSION

Intergenerational relationships play a key role in shaping individuals and communities, fostering understanding and contributing to the continuity of cultural values across generations. During this survey, we delved into different aspects of intergenerational relationships and explored their importance, challenges and potential impact on social cohesion. As we conclude, it is clear that these relationships are complex and multifaceted, influenced by cultural, societal, and individual factors.

One of the key themes that emerged is the importance of communication in intergenerational relationships. Effective communication serves as a cornerstone for understanding, bridging generational gaps and strengthening a sense of connection. The exchange of ideas, experiences and wisdom between different age groups not only enriches individual lives, but also contributes to the collective knowledge of society. Fostering open dialogue and active listening becomes essential in overcoming potential misunderstandings and fostering empathy across generations.

Furthermore, the role of technology in shaping intergenerational relationships cannot be neglected. As rapid technological advances continue to change the way individuals interact, the digital divide between generations can present challenges. But when approached thoughtfully, technology has the potential to facilitate intergenerational connections and provide platforms for shared experiences and mutual learning.

Another essential aspect is the interplay of tradition and modernity within intergenerational relations. For the healthy development of these relationships, it is essential to find a balance between the preservation of cultural heritage and the acceptance of social change. While tradition provides a sense of continuity and identity, adapting to the evolving dynamics of society ensures relevance and inclusiveness across generations.

Challenges in intergenerational relationships also stem from differences in values, attitudes and lifestyle choices. Recognizing and respecting these differences is essential to promoting harmony. Intergenerational conflicts can arise when expectations clash, but through mutual understanding and compromise, these conflicts can be overcome, leading to stronger and more resilient relationships.

The influence of intergenerational relationships goes beyond the individual and affects social structures and norms. Policies that encourage intergenerational interactions and support programs that bridge generational gaps contribute to the overall well-being of communities. Recognizing each generation's valuable contribution and creating opportunities for collaboration can lead to a more cohesive and vibrant society.

When we think about intergenerational relationships, it is clear that their importance goes beyond family ties. They shape the narratives of communities and serve as a conduit for the transmission of knowledge, values and cultural heritage. Nurturing these relationships requires intentional effort with a commitment to understanding, appreciation, and adaptability.

Intergenerational relationships are a dynamic tapestry woven from threads of communication, technology, tradition and adaptation. They are necessary to promote a sense of continuity, promote mutual understanding and enrich the structure of society. Embracing diversity across generations and recognizing the interconnectedness of past, present and future lays the foundation for a harmonious and resilient community. As we navigate the complexities of the modern world, the strength of our intergenerational bonds will undoubtedly play a vital role in shaping the legacy we leave for generations to come.